Te Rongoa Maori

Maori Medicine

Te Rongoa Maori

Maori Medicine

P.M.E. Williams

REED

Illustration Acknowledgements

The cover painting of lacebark is by E. Blumhardt. The illustrations reproduced in the text include paintings by Fanny Osborne and E. Blumhardt and etchings by S. Parkinson. The Osborne painting of pirita is owned by Mrs G.C. Haden; the Osborne painting of tataramoa is owned by Mrs S. Nicol; they are reproduced by kind permission. The remainder of the illustrations are reproduced by kind permission of the copyright holder, Auckland Institute and Museum.

Published 1996 by Reed Books, a division of Reed Publishing (NZ) Ltd, 39 Rawene Rd, Birkenhead, Auckland. Associated companies, branches and representatives throughout the world.

ISBN 0 7900 0510 7

Designed by Clair Stutton and Zoë Nash

Printed in Hong Kong by Dah Hua Printing Press Co., Ltd

Reprinted 1999

Dedication

Dedicated to the Ngapuhi people
Ki taku iwi Maori, whakapai, whakapai, whakapai

Acknowledgments

My thanks go to Rachel Hind, who typed the manuscript, and Heather Ayrton for her invaluable help and advice. Without their help and that of the Tai Tokerau Trust this book would never have been started. I thank also my old friends who shared their knowledge with me and taught me all I know.

Publisher's note

The author and publisher advise that this book is not intended as a practical guide for prescribing medicines or for curing sicknesses. Neither the author nor the publisher can accept responsibility for the popular remedies that have been recorded here.

Contents

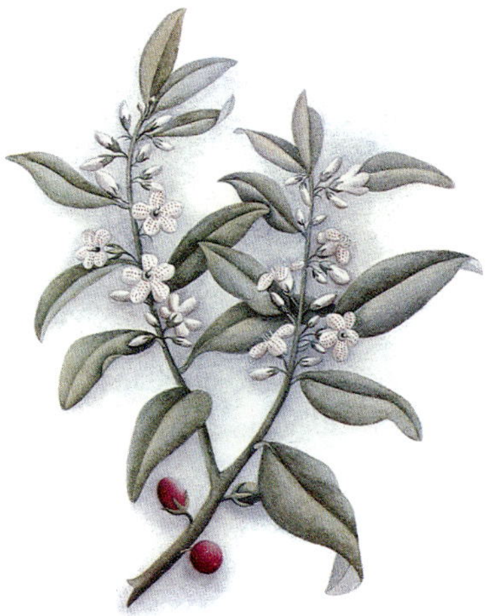

Ngaio

Myoporum laetum (p.47)

F. Osborne

Foreword

Publication of his observations of the use by Maori of plant material for medicinal purposes is a triumph for Pip Williams in his ninety-third year.

As a pharmacist in Kaikohe serving a large section of the mid North during the 1930s Depression, and during and after the Second World War, Pip Williams had first-hand experience of the lore and the financial constraints that gave reason for the use of Maori medicines.

The timing of publication is significant when health services are being restructured and more Maori (and some Pakeha) are returning to the bush for the cures for many of their ills.

Underlying the author's knowledge of medicines both pharmaceutical and Maori, either from plants or the influence of the tohunga, is his long association with orthodox health practice. The latter culminated in his chairmanship of the Northland Hospital Board for 24 years and ten years as a member of the New Zealand Hospital Boards' Association.

Of equal importance is his knowledge and love of the Maori people.

Pip Williams makes no recommendations but indicates which plants were used for various problems, colourfully interspersing his notes with anecdotal evidence.

Heather Ayrton

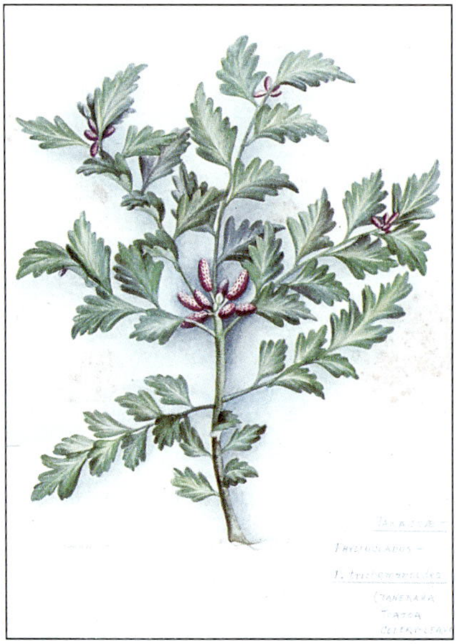

Tanekaha

Celery pine

Phyllocladus trichomanoides (p.67)

F. Osborne

Introduction

My Life in Maori Health

After receiving a very good education at Napier Boys' High School I started my pharmacy career at Knights Pharmacy in Hastings. I spent the next 14 years in Hawke's Bay, first as an apprentice then as a locum assistant manager in Dannevirke. During that time I learned very little about Maori medicine. I had heard about the heavy bruising of All Black George Nepia and his visit to Mrs Paewai Snr (see page 31), and when visiting my folks at Te Awanga did witness a drowning accident in which the victim, a boy, was suspended by his feet over a smoky fire until he sneezed, got rid of the water and recovered.

When I went north to Kaikohe, however, I passed into a new world as far as medicine was concerned. I found that my customers made their own concoctions and were very much under the influence of the tohunga, there being only one available doctor — Dr G.M. Smith — who visited once a week. I therefore became the 'doctor', vet, social worker and friend. Even so it was quite a while before the local people had enough faith in me to tell me what they were using.

Prior to the coming of the Pakeha, Maori lost their teeth through chewing fern root, had back deterioration from carrying rocks and wood, and were lucky if they lived beyond 35 years of age. What a 'party' for the tohunga! He had his own methods of treatment. For example, he and an ailing patient would wade waist deep into a stream (no fear of hypothermia) then, holding high some puha or other greenery, the tohunga would wave it over his patient from right to left. This would dispatch the devil by way of the ara atua or way of the god. Placing karamu or *Coprosma* branches on the patient's body was an alternative way of driving out a devil or evil spirit.

Having learnt of some of the traditional remedies, I am inclined to believe missionaries such as William Colenso who thought it highly unlikely that Maori used any internal medicine before the arrival of Europeans. With the Europeans, however, there also came a number of problems for Maori — health problems which took years to cure. Whalers brought tuberculosis, venereal disease and measles, which affected especially Maori women with whom they had intercourse.

The early missionaries found that Maori were fascinated by the mixture of water and Epsom salts. Their problems were due mostly to stomach disorders, constipation and dysentery. Whenever Pakeha medicine failed to cure immediately, Maori went back to the tohunga who treated them with a lot of karakia and his own secret concoctions. Maori believed that it took a Maori medicine to treat a Maori.

During the 30 to 40 years I was lecturing on Te Rongoa Maori and listening to Maori, I was surprised by the lack of knowledge of New Zealand trees and plants among audiences, whether people belonged to service clubs, garden clubs, or were university students. City residents were the least knowledgeable.

Te Rongoa Maori aims, in an informal way, to introduce a particular class of native flora utilised by Maori — plants and trees that over the years have been found to have therapeutic benefits for a variety of health problems.

Most of the information here comprises what I have been told by kuia and my own observations. Maori in earlier times knew about trees and plants and their medicinal uses but had no knowledge of pharmacology, and I have just recorded what older Maori taught me. The remedies are those I have copied from my notes written 40 years ago, but I take no responsibility for their efficacy. That doesn't mean, however, that one cannot listen and learn, and when antibiotics prove no longer successful, who knows, we may return to natural remedies. The kuia and kaumatua to whom I listened are now long gone but their knowledge survives.

Many people, both Pakeha and Maori, have asked me also to include other observations and incidents related to plants, that refer to intriguing 'handy-hints' rather than medicinal uses. I hope that such details may provide some light-hearted interest.

God bless, and pleasant reading.

To my Maori friends, Ma te atua koutou katoa i tiaki.

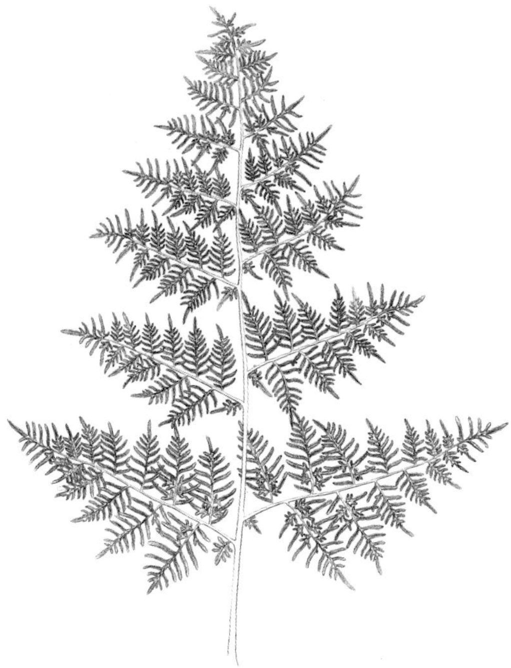

S. Parkinson
engraving

Bracken

Rahurahu or Rarahu

Pteridium esculentum

Bracken fern is widespread throughout New Zealand in open areas and in forest margins. One friend, Bill Wihongi, our paramount chief, told me that the best place to collect fern root was from a garden on the edge of Lake Omapere.

The thin, coarse roots were pounded and then boiled or baked; this food was a staple of the Maori diet, and may have been responsible for the deterioration in their teeth.

The boiled or baked roots were also fed to infants; in more modern times, cow's milk was added. One young mother told me this mixture had been better than Glaxo.

Other uses included chewing the raw roots to treat dysentery, and eating cooked bracken root before putting to sea in order to prevent sea sickness.

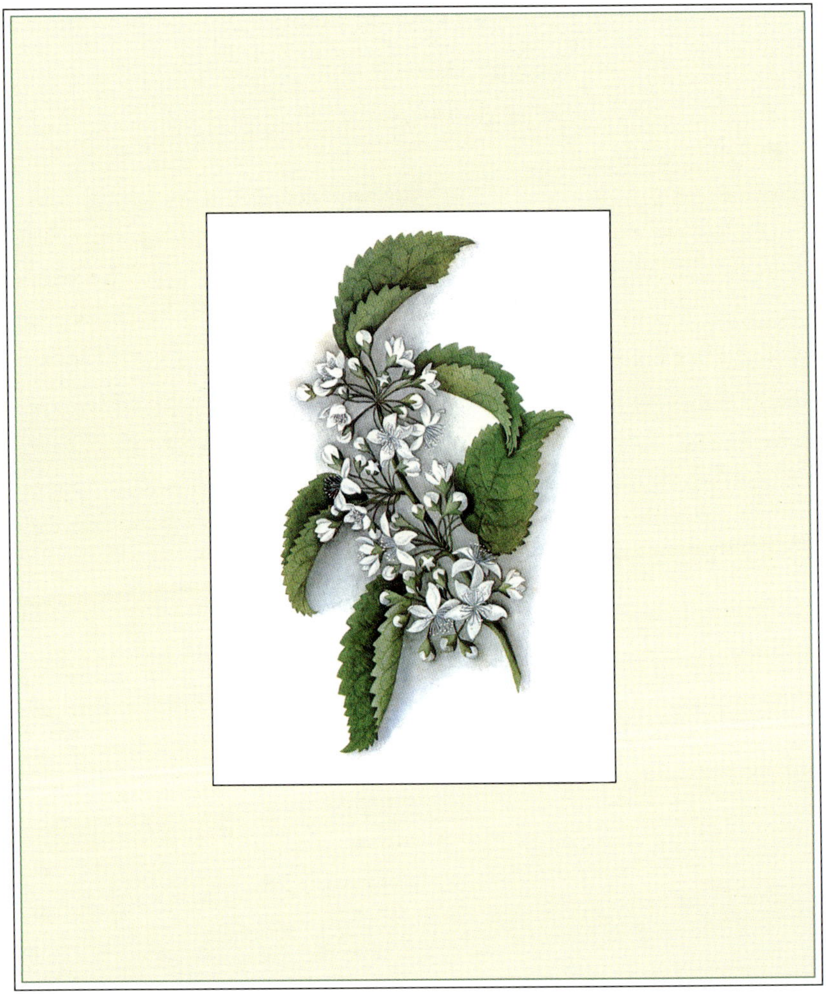

F. Osborne

Hoiheri, Houhere

Lacebark

Hoheria populnea

Hoiheri is better known as lacebark because of the lace-patterned layers that form its inner bark. In my garden, in a good season, I have seen a tree covered in lovely white flowers. Maori women in Kaikohe used to make beautiful evening purses from the lace-like inner bark. I was most impressed with these and other delicate articles they made.

An infusion of the bark of houhere was taken for colds and, when soaked in cold water to form a jelly, was used by old people to treat sore eyes. As with many other small trees, the bark was also used as a poultice. The inner bark, prepared with the sap of flax leaves, was applied to treat burns.

Kahikatea

White pine

Dacrycarpus dacrydioides

The very picturesque kahikatea is New Zealand's tallest tree and is found throughout the country, particularly in swampy conditions.

I've been told that short branches were boiled and the vapour inhaled. I know of one kuia who recommended an infusion of kahikatea leaves as the best tonic she knew. The leaves were also used to treat kidney and other urinary problems. To relieve bruising, bushmen boiled the leaves in water and applied them with a rag or moss.

Karaka

Corynocarpus laevigatus

Karaka grows extensively around the coast where it is admired for its glossy leaves and yellow berries. As it is able to withstand strong winds, karaka is used extensively as hedging.

The berries, or rather the seeds, are highly prized as a food source by Maori. Because the seeds are poisonous in their raw state, however, they are boiled for eight to ten hours then put in a kete or flax kit and left in fresh running water for a couple of days. Children then eat the yellow pulp. When dried, the seeds become quite palatable to chew and are known as Maori peanuts.

The leaves were used as a poultice on wounds, with the upper surface of the leaf placed downwards; the rougher lower surface actually draws out any pus.

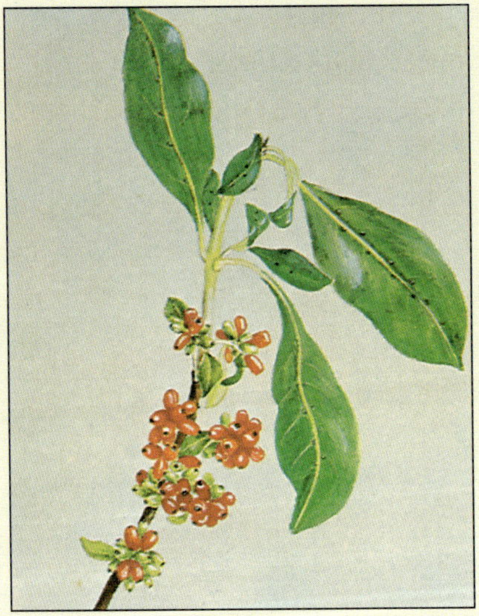

Coprosma robusta

E. Blumhardt

Karamu

Coprosma spp.

There are over 40 species of *Coprosma* in New Zealand. The glossy-leaved karamu (C. *robusta*) is widespread in the main islands in forests and forest margins.

A compress of the leaves of karamu was applied to relieve aches and pains. Cuts, sores and bruises were treated with a decoction of the leaves in water, and the sap was applied for scabies.

For internal applications, a liquor was made by boiling karamu shoots in water and used for kidney and bladder complaints.

I believe that an infusion of the leaves was also used to reduce fever but I have no verification of this.

I do know that the tohunga incorporated karamu in some of his rites and karakia to expel an evil spirit or demon from a patient.

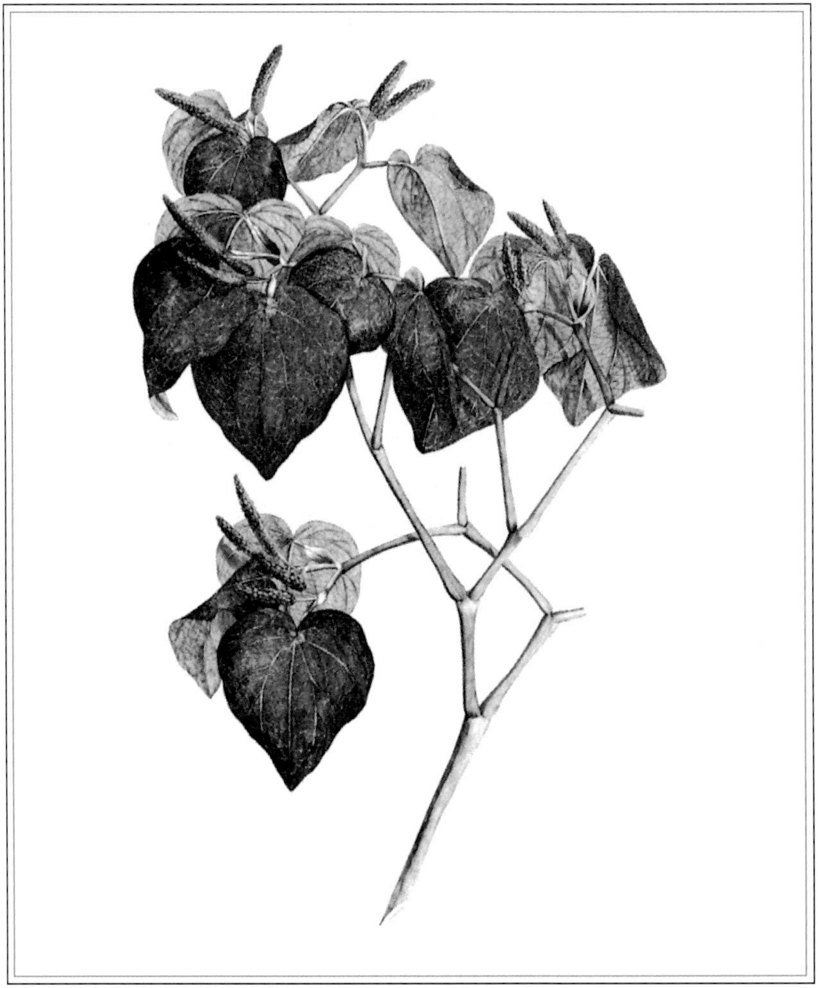

S. Parkinson

Kawakawa

Maori pepper tree

Macropiper excelsum

Kawakawa grows everywhere around the coast. In fact there is so much of it around the Bay of Islands that a town there bears its name.

The pepper aspect of kawakawa excited the kidneys and bowels and was used by older men as an aphrodisiac to renew their youth. A decoction of the leaves is still used in the treatment of boils and for kidney troubles. I have also been told that an infusion of the leaves was a blood purifier and definitely would cure paipai (a skin disease common in young Maori). Kawakawa was also used to treat gonorrhoea.

Many tales have been told about kawakawa's medicinal values, but usually it is used to relieve toothache (by chewing the leaves) or a swollen face.

Kiekie

Freycinetia banksii

Kiekie is a fast-growing climbing shrub found in most Northland bush areas and in the Auckland region but is less plentiful further south. The fruit has a tropical appearance with its 8–10 centimetre-long green spike surrounded by white bracts. Kiekie is related to pandanus which is used extensively in the Pacific Islands for weaving, and, in New Zealand, Maori wove baskets from the leaves.

More important, however, is the flower or fruit (tawhara), which ripens in October when it is the size of a small cabbage and is very sweet and palatable. Provided you get ahead of the rats and possums, you will enjoy what is a real treat, but the fruit lasts for only a few weeks. I knew of one Maori family who every October had a day in the bush gathering and eating tawhara straight from the bush, because unfortunately it does not keep. Being so sweet, tawhara must be the best of our native-bush fruits. The fruit is also slightly laxative, which is its most likely medicinal use.

Kohekohe

Native cedar

Dysoxylum spectabile

Kohekohe is my favourite tree. It is found in bush mainly near the coast, and grows very well here at Paihia. The seedling is often mistaken for puriri. Kohekohe must have a tropical origin because I know of no other instance where the florets grow directly from the mature wood, followed by the berries. Kaikohe women and children lived on these berries in the bush. I have obtained a kohekohe bole from an old tree damaged by the wind, and intend to have a table made from it.

An infusion of young kohekohe bark was used as a tonic by bushmen for stomach troubles. Infusion of both the leaves and bark was taken whenever blood was involved. For tuberculosis an infusion of young bark (in water) was a great help in relieving spitting, and in treating lung haemorrhage and women's menstrual discomfort it had no equal.

Some kuia have told me that their parents had used poultices of boiled leaves to treat gonorrhoea and other similar problems that were a legacy of the whalers. I know a poultice was also used for many other diseases, as well as for bleeding piles, kidney complaints and menstrual disorders.

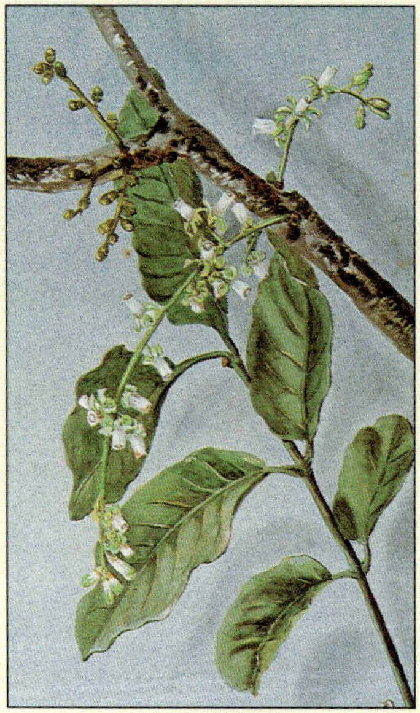

Kohekohe

Native cedar

Dysoxylum spectabile

E. Blumhardt

How Kaikohe got its name

While the menfolk of Hakina Pa (now Kaikohe) were away at Lake Omapere gathering food — taro, fern root, kakahi and eels from the lake — Ngati Whatua from Kaipara (Dargaville) attacked. Under the guidance of a relative of the Ngapuhi chief Hongi Hika, the women and children of the pa escaped into the bush on Toka Rei Reia, now known as Monument Hill. There they hid among the kohekohe trees and lived on the berries from the trees.

When the men collecting food heard about the Ngati Whatua attack they returned to the pa and found the chief of the invaders on his own, away from his warriors who were eating around their fires. They captured him and made him promise to leave immediately and never attack the pa again. When the women and children returned they told how they had lived on the berries of the kohekohe, hence the settlement's name: kai (food) of the kohekohe — Kaikohe.

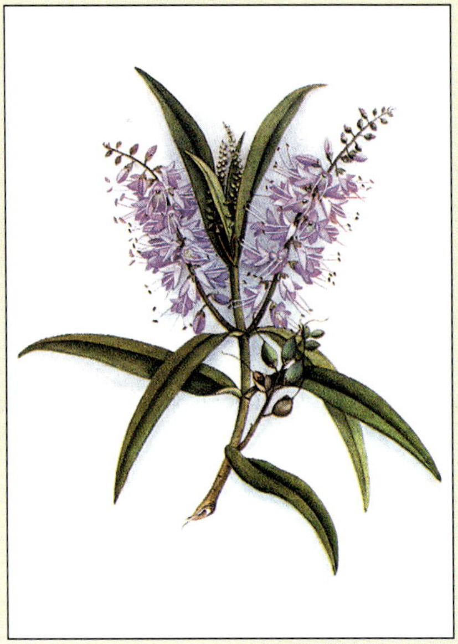

Hebe macrocarpa

F. Osborne

Koromiko

Hebe

Hebe spp.

Many species of this beautiful and valuable shrub grow in New Zealand gardens.

Hebe was a plant used for vapour baths; the bruised leaves were heated and used as a poultice for ulcers; and liquid from the boiled leaves was used as a gargle.

However, it was as a cure for diarrhoea and dysentery that hebe was used by both Maori and Pakeha. Although when one considers the simple staple diet of the early settlers and Maori people, it is a wonder that stomach disorders did appear regularly, be it diarrhoea, dysentery or constipation. I often wonder whether hygiene had anything to do with these health problems

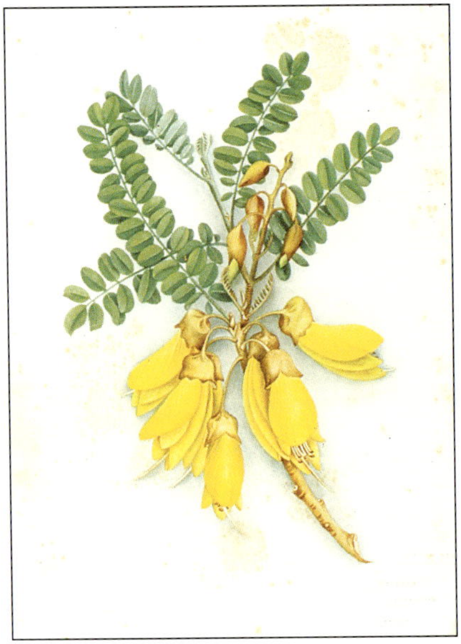

F. Osborne

Kowhai

Sophora microphylla

Because of its beautiful yellow flowers, Maori often referred to the kowhai to signify the colour 'yellow'.

Kowhai was used for itch and other skin diseases. An infusion of the bark and some other plants, such as koromiko and manuka seeds, was taken as a drink for internal pains.

There is a saying in the Bay of Islands: 'When the kowhai is in flower, the fish are up the Waitangi.'

The Nepia story

I was playing football in Hastings when the 1924–25 All Blacks returned from England. George Nepia had come home with bruises all over his body and the Hawke's Bay physiotherapist Mr Hildebrant said he wasn't to play that season, so he went for a holiday to Dannevirke, to the home of his friend Lui Paewai. Lui's mother said she would cure him. She broke a bottle and with the sharp edges lightly scratched the bruises and blood parts. She then made George get into a warm to hot bath prepared with kowhai bark. This procedure was repeated for a few days and, a week or so later, George played football again. Remarkable but true.

Kumarahou

Gumdigger's soap

Pomaderris kumaraho

Kumarahou grows everywhere on the gumfields of the North and in the scrub on the edges of roads. The shrub displays a profusion of golden flowers during spring.

Ask anyone in the North, 'What do you know of Maori medicine?' and they will immediately say, 'Kumarahou, great stuff.'

It would appear that kumarahou was used internally for virtually everything: coughs, colds, asthma, bronchitis. A liquor of the boiled leaves was taken for these ailments. One kuia told me the infusion was good for the kidneys and was an effective tonic.

Mahoe

Whiteywood

Melicytus ramiflorus

Mahoe is widespread in New Zealand and is one of the most common small trees in forests and scrublands. It has lovely purple berries. We have a small settlement in the Bay of Islands called Oramahoe.

Mahoe had several external uses, including treating burns with an application of the teased inner bark. Rheumaticky joints were bathed in an infusion of the leaves (as strong as for regular tea). Skin problems, especially scabies, were treated with boiled leaves compressed into a bandage.

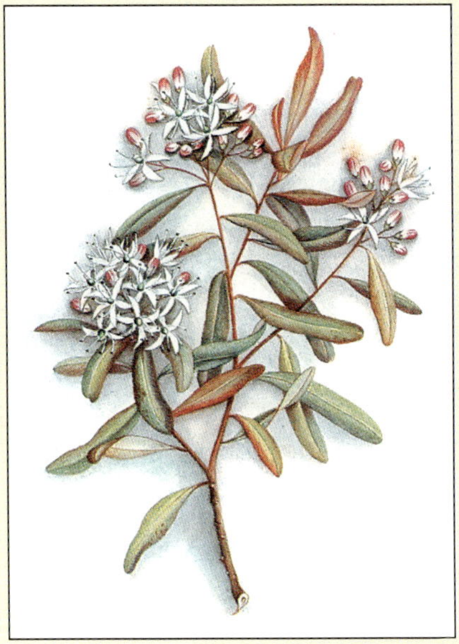

F. Osborne

Mairehau

Phebalium nudum

Mairehau is found in kauri forests and manuka scrubland. It is a graceful, much-branched shrub with beautiful white flowers and an aromatic perfume. The perfume comes from the leaves which are dotted with oil glands.

Maori used to rub the fragrant leaves on their bodies. Mairehau leaves were also used in burials. When a body was being prepared it was wrapped in a mat with the leaves then buried or, in Kaikohe, it was lowered down the vent of Putahi, an extinct volcano near the shores of Lake Omapere.

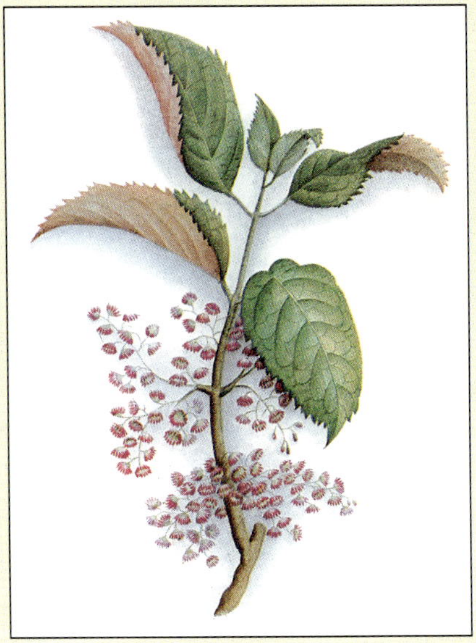

F. Osborne

Makomako

Wineberry

Aristotelia serrata

Makomako is an attractive small tree common throughout the country. It is often transplanted to gardens as a sapling.

The bark was used in a bath for rheumatism. The leaves were boiled and the liquid then applied to sore eyes and boils. The boiled leaves themselves were applied to burns.

Although in earlier times Maori did not make use of the berries, European settlers soon got the idea of making wine from the juice extracted from the berries, hence the tree's common English name.

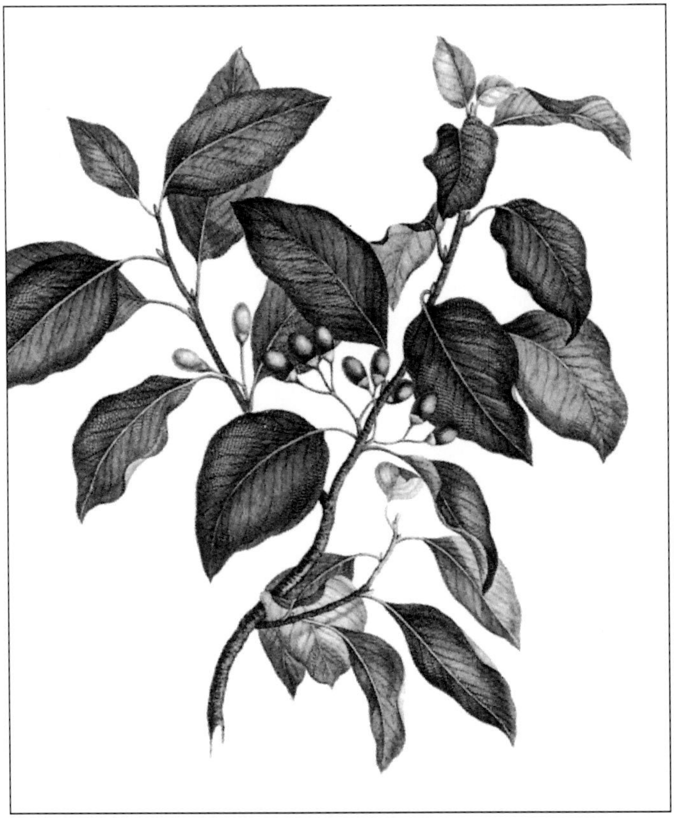

S. Parkinson
engraving

Mangeao

Litsea calicaris

Mangeao is a lovely tree that grows only sparsely in the North.

I believe it was used in midwifery to facilitate the delivery of the baby, but I found it also had other uses. A decoction was taken as a drink for biliousness and rheumatism.

Like miro and kauri, mangeao wood was used to make yokes for bullock teams. Being light and tough it was much prized. I've often thought it would make a good cricket bat as it would never split.

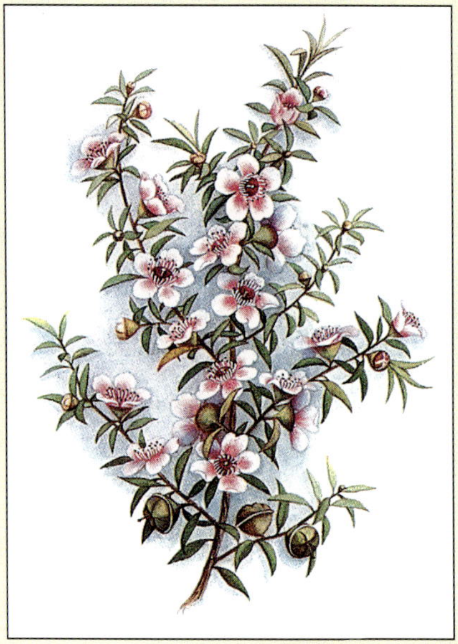

Manuka

F. Osborne

Manuka
Red ti/tea tree
Leptospermum scoparium

Kanuka
White ti/tea tree
Leptospermum ericoides

Manuka and kanuka are handsome shrubs that are found throughout New Zealand, though the mature kanuka can become a tall spreading tree. In Northland both species are known as manuka. They have many uses, the earliest written recorded use being that by Captain Cook, who had the leaves infused with totara leaves as a drink to cure his crew of scurvy. Early settlers brewed the leaves as a substitute for tea, hence the common English name.

An infusion of the leaves was also used as a drink to treat kidney and bladder complaints and to reduce fever in children. It was often used to ease coughing in adults. A decoction of the bark was another cure for diarrhoea and dysentery, but it is the capsules or seeds with which I am most acquainted. They seem to have had many uses. When chewed they were universally successful in curing stomach complaints. I was also told that a poultice of the crushed and boiled seeds was effective in healing an open wound. A decoction of the leaves and bark was also applied to ease pain.

A small industry has been started on the East Coast to extract the oil of these species which is said to be effective against some diseases where antibiotics have proved unsuccessful. We have not heard the last of these trees, and further research is called for.

Matai

Black pine

Prumnopitys taxifolia

Matai is a tall forest tree found throughout New Zealand. It is prized by bushmen as it is suitable for milling and makes sturdy flooring. The roots are used in open fires.

Bushmen have told me how much they have enjoyed matai 'beer', a refreshing sap collected by drilling the base of old trees with an auger. In fact the beer seems to be what the bushmen remember most! Matai beer did have a medicinal use — as a disinfectant in the treatment of consumption.

Matipo

Mapau

Myrsine australis

Matipo or mapau is a shrub or small tree found around the coast but seldom inland. I have some very attractive specimens growing in my bush.

The kuia tell me that the liquid taken from the boiled leaves was effective in alleviating toothache, but I think kawakawa was more popular.

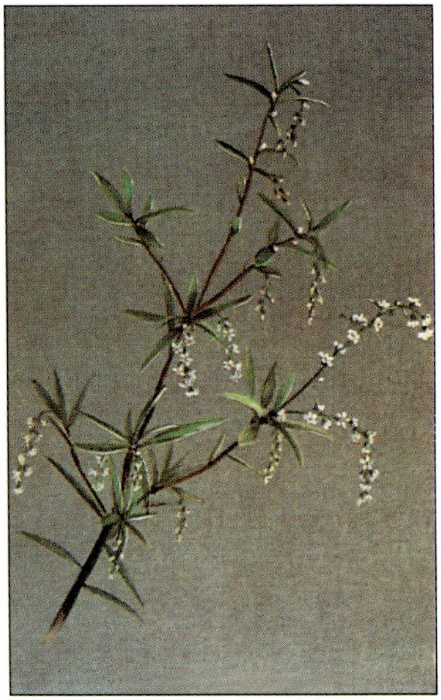

Leucopogon fasciculatus

E. Blumhardt

Mingimingi, Taumingi, Tumingi

Cyathodes juniperina / Leucopogon fasciculatus

Mingimingi is the popular name for both a small-leaved shrub (*Cyathodes juniperina*) and a small tree (*Leucopogon fasciculatus*) that are plentiful in the North.

A decoction of the leaves boiled in water was taken as a drink for kidney complaints and asthma. According to bushmen, this liquid, like that from toot, was also used as a dressing for septic wounds. The decoction was used as well by women for menstrual difficulties, and I have heard of it being used for headaches and even influenza.

Miro

Brown pine

Prumnopitys ferruginea

Miro is a tall tree found in most of New Zealand's forests, and is especially attractive to pigeons because of its purplish-coloured berries.

An infusion of the leaves and bark was used by bushmen as an antiseptic and insecticide. I don't know how effective this was, but a few people were definitely using it when I first went to Kaikohe.

The gum from the bark was applied to wounds and ulcers, and an infusion of leaves and bark was taken to treat gonorrhoea and stomach aches.

Ngaio

Myoporum laetum

Ngaio is a small shrub or tree found around the coast (see illustration on page 8). It is poisonous to animals, so most farmers — who can put up with sandflies so long as their cattle are safe — have cleared their farms of ngaio.

The sticky black shoots, or an infusion of the leaves, were rubbed over the body to keep sandflies and mosquitoes at bay. If one had a lot of dental trouble the inner bark was rubbed on the gums and chewed. I believe that a weak infusion was also applied to treat eczema in babies.

My brother once used a poultice of leaves on a wounded horse with great drawing effect — he said it was strong enough to lift the mortgage off the farm!

Nikau

Rhopalostylis sapida

The nikau — one of only two native palms — is a lovely ornamental tree that is very graceful when fully grown.

The inner pith in the bulbous part below the leaves has a mild laxative quality. An infusion of this was taken as a drink to ease childbirth. Such an infusion was also used to treat diarrhoea and dysentery.

The nikau provided a very valuable building material for the Maori. The leaves or fronds were used as a thatch on the manuka framework of the whare, resulting in a warm, dry shelter.

Piripiri

Bididbid/i

Acaena spp.

Piripiri is the bane of all sheep farmers where it is prevalent. The seeds attach themselves to the sheep's wool and can damage the fleece.

A decoction of the leaves was taken as a tonic and used for kidney and bladder problems. It was also taken as a treatment for venereal disease.

I heard from one kuia that an application of the infusion was very good for an old skin disease generally referred to as 'hakihaki', which has more sores and is more extensive a rash than paipai (a skin disease caused by lice).

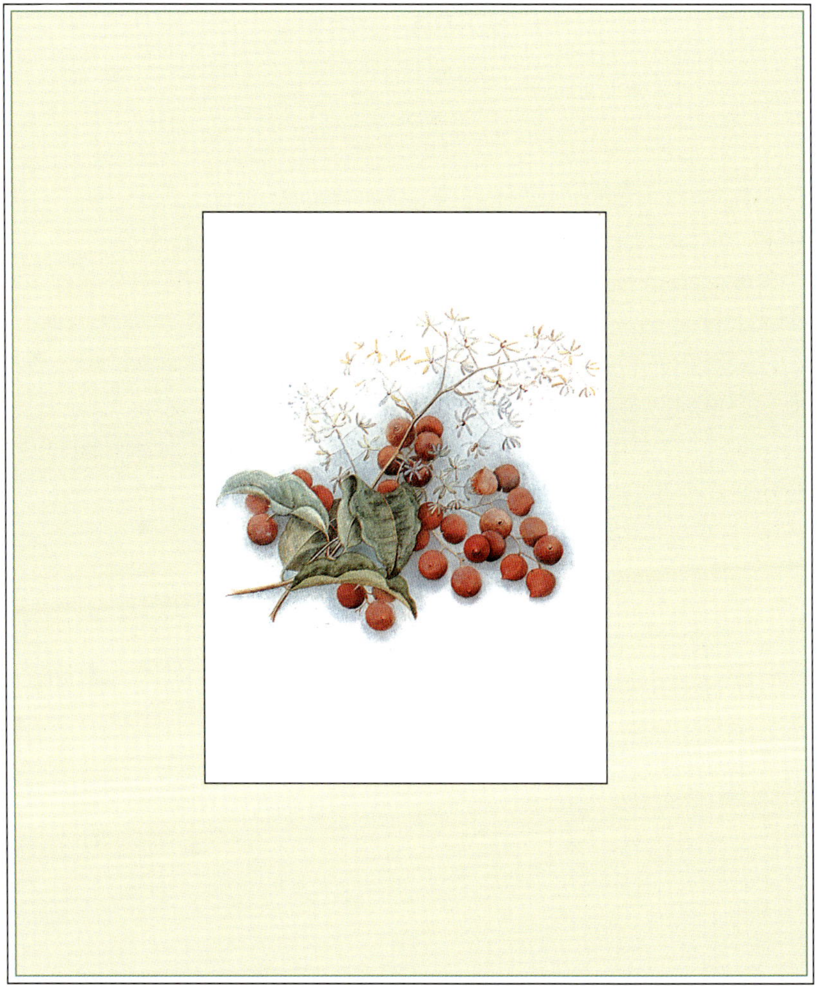

F. Osborne

Pirita

Supplejack

Ripogonum scandens

Pirita is a climbing woody plant which forms a mass of twisting stems. It is widespread in lowland forests.

Shoots were cut and the sap applied to cuts and scrapes.

A cold infusion of the leaves was taken as a drink to treat rheumatism, as was a decoction of the roots which was also used as a universal remedy for skin troubles, bowel complaints, fever and general weakness. One kuia told me it was used to relieve syphilis as well. It is reported that the stems were used externally in the treatment of venereal disease but as I had no patients with such illness, I could not prove this.

Pohatu

Wild turnip

Brassica rapa

The sap of this plant combined with the sap of puwha was taken as a drink to correct any bleeding after childbirth. I cannot add more to this except to say that the kuia who were looking after the patients told me it worked.

Ponga
Siver fern
Cyathea dealbata

Mamaku
Black tree fern
Cyathea medullaris

Ponga and mamaku are common throughout most of New Zealand, but are also known by different names in the North, such as korau, which is another name for mamaku.

In midwifery, young fronds were heated and used for poulticing a mother's inflamed breasts and when boiled the liquid was taken as a drink to help expel the afterbirth.

Bushmen have told me that a poultice made from the heated fronds helped to cure sores and wounds.

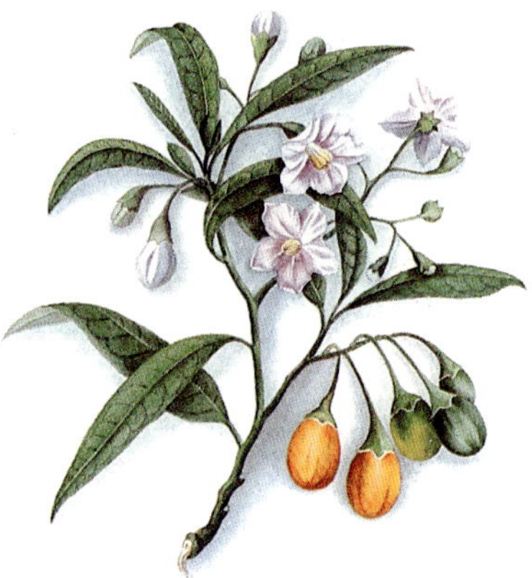

Solanum aviculare

F. Osborne

Poroporo, Kohoho

Nightshade

Solanum aviculare, S. laciniatum

Poroporo is a small shrub found everywhere, especially around the coast.

The leaves when boiled and used as a vegetable are a great source of iron.

The inner bark and leaves were prepared as a liquid or as a poultice to treat various skin diseases, successfully I believe. They were also used in the same way for ulcers.

Puha, Puwha

Sow thistle

Sonchus oleraceus

Puha is a vegetable plant growing throughout New Zealand and is used as such by Maori. I eat it myself frequently and Maori friends visit regularly to collect a meal from my garden. Pork bones and puha make up one of their favourite dishes. I believe Captain Cook had puha boiled to be eaten by crew members affected by scurvy.

Puha was also prepared as a drink for stomach ailments, boils and carbuncles, and for women giving birth to expel the placenta and to ease any long haemorrhaging afterwards. The milky sap from crushed puha leaves is used by both Maori and Pakeha to cure warts, especially in children. Rich in iron, puha is also used as a tonic.

Another traditional use of puha is made by tohunga in various rites.

Pukatea

Laurelia novae-zelandiae

Pukatea is a stately forest tree, found throughout most of the country. I once had a pukatea growing near a spring in a swampy area.

To alleviate toothache, my neighbours used to obtain a liquid by steeping the inner bark in hot water and applying this to the painful area. I think they also used to apply the liquid to some skin complaints. The liquid was used to treat chronic ulcers as well. In earlier times the decoction was used as a lotion to treat syphilis.

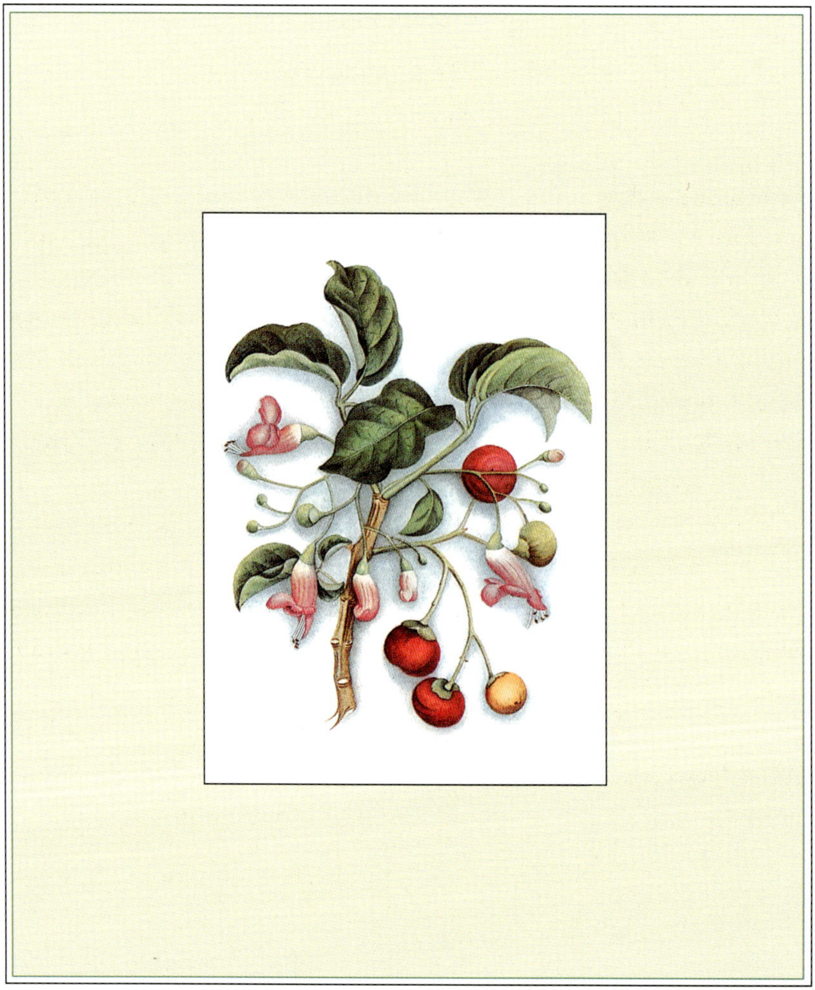

F. Osborne

Puriri

New Zealand oak

Vitex lucens

Puriri grows widely in Northland but this beautiful, spreading hardwood tree does not occur in any abundance further south. Some lovely puriri grow around Waimate North.

The liquor from leaves boiled in water was applied to relieve sprains, backache and ulcers. One Sunday morning a neighbour visited me and asked if he could have some puriri leaves. He had an ulcer which developed while he'd been in the desert with the Maori Battalion. He'd tried plenty of doctors and, while it wasn't getting any worse, neither was it getting any better. He asked for some blue-gum leaves as well. He went on home, boiled up the leaves, got some cotton wool and made a compress which he put on the ulcer. When I left Kaikohe a month later there was a light skin over the ulcer. Whether it lasted or not I don't know because having left Kaikohe for Paihia I lost touch and he has since died.

I have also heard of an infusion of the leaves being taken as a drink to treat kidney complaints.

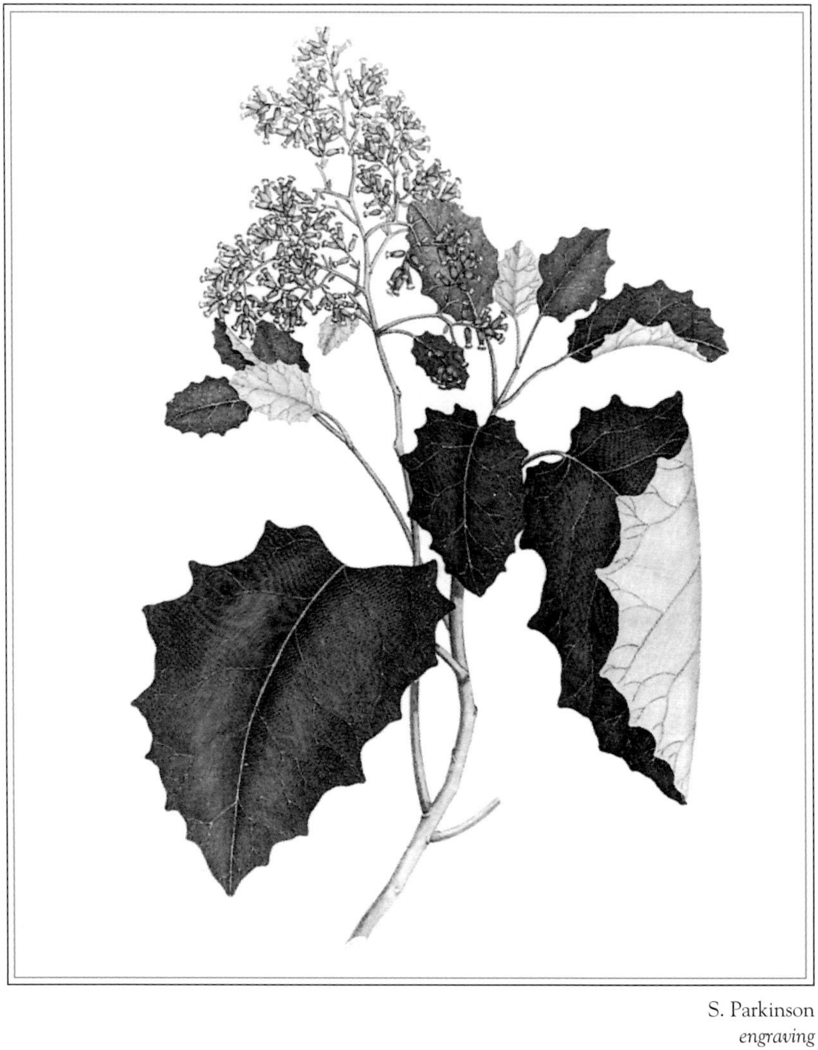

S. Parkinson
engraving

Rangiora, Pukapuka, Wharangi

Brachyglottis repanda

Rangiora is a shrub with an attractive small flower that is found in most places in the North Island.

The leaves and gum from an incision in the bark were chewed together to eliminate bad breath but never swallowed as the plant is poisonous. I noticed this practice was popular with old men.

As with karaka leaves, the smooth side of rangiora leaves healed sores and ulcers, while the rough under-side was effective as a drawing agent.

Rata

Metrosideros robusta

Rata is found everywhere in the North and South Islands, although the white variety is not as plentiful as the red. Usually rata begins life as an epiphyte growing on another tree which eventually encloses the host and forms a tall hardwood specimen. In recent years the rata has become a prime food source of possums, which have destroyed large numbers of this magnificent tree.

Bushmen cut the young aerial roots and drank the plentiful and refreshing sap that exuded.

An early-settler farmer friend of mine told me the sap was very effective for eye troubles and any cuts. He also told me his Maori workmen applied it to treat ringworm.

Raupo

Bulrush

Typha orientalis

Raupo is a reed found in marshy places throughout New Zealand.

The fluffy part of the seeds was applied to wounds, old ulcers and sores to keep them free of dirt and dust. In midwifery, the root or rhizome was boiled with the roots of the flax plant and the liquid given as a drink to help expel the afterbirth.

Raupo's greatest use, however, was as housing material for the side walls of a nikau whare.

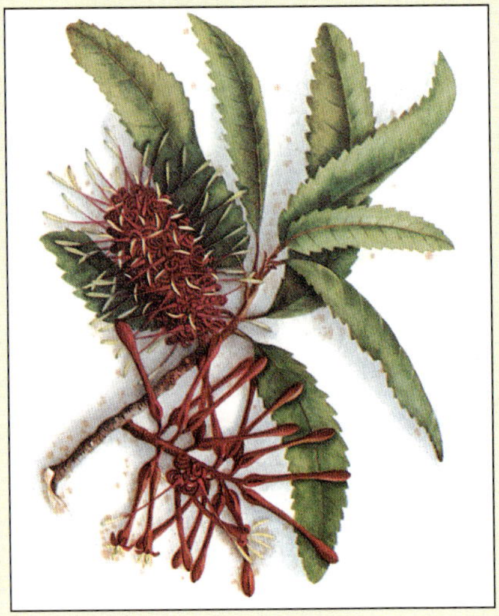

F. Osborne

Rewarewa

Honeysuckle

Knightia excelsa

Rewarewa is common in the North Island and the top of the South Island. When fully grown it is a fine tree, with lovely mottled wood. After a bush burn it is the first tree to appear.

The inner bark was applied in its raw state by bushmen to stem the bloodflow from cuts; it was also used as a bandage.

Rimuroa, Rimurapa, Rimurehia

Bull kelp/Seaweeds

Durvillaea antarctica and other species

Rimuroa is the usual spelling of one of the many seaweeds in New Zealand waters.

One day when looking out my window at Paihia, I could see a boat on the Brampton (a shoal), and boys diving. Being curious I decided to find out what was happening. I was told they were after seaweed, which they were selling to make agar. After further enquiries of older Maori I was told that rimuroa was roasted and eaten to treat worms and serious skin diseases.

A Rotary student once told me that in Japan she used to eat candied seaweed as we would eat a sweet, and a friend's mother used to make a lovely custard out of seaweed.

I have seen bull kelp hung outside the door of a whare as a barometer or rain gauge. It was dry when the weather was fine and swelled when rain was coming.

Tanekaha

Celery pine

Phyllocladus trichomanoides

Tanekaha is a very neat forest tree found in both islands (see illustration on page 10). When small, it makes an attractive garden specimen.

Although in coastal areas the tannic acid in the inner bark has been used for dysentery I have never heard of it being used as such by Kaikohe people.

Tanekaha does, however, have assorted non-medicinal uses. A very young tanekaha tied in a knot and left to grow will make a fine walking stick with a round handle. Tanekaha also makes good fishing rods. I once found a nice sapling, trimmed it and left it in my creek for a couple of weeks. In fact I quite forgot about it. I then dried it and placed it in a pipe which I filled with sump oil from my car. I left it for three months and when I fitted it up with a reel and fair leads, I had the best deep-sea rod anyone could wish for. It lasted for years. A well-known deep-sea skipper told me he always used tanekaha rods in the early days, but he used the top of the tree, trimmed it to size and left it in a stream for a couple of weeks. He then painted it with raw linseed oil and left it for a week — result, a wonderful rod. Tanekaha was also used to dye ropes and nets.

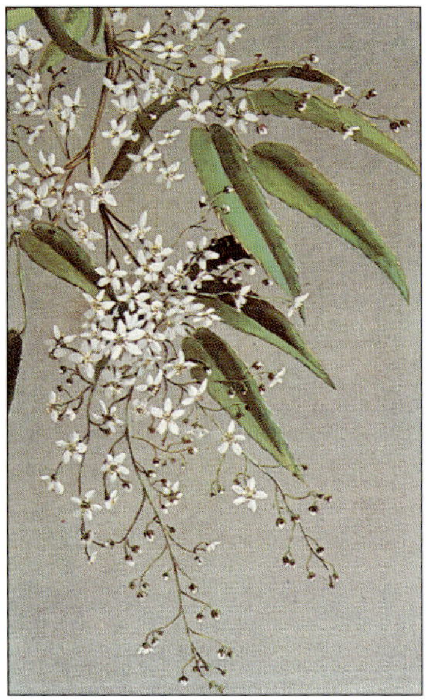

Rubus cissoides

E. Blumhardt

Tataramoa

Bush lawyer

Rubus spp.

Tataramoa is a vine found in the bush in most parts of New Zealand, and its white flowers are conspicuous in spring. The vine will cling to anyone brushing against it, hence the name 'bush lawyer'.

To ease the pains of constipation, a liquid of the boiled bark was drunk. An alternative treatment was to eat the young leaves. I was told that an infusion of the root bark helped to cure diarrhoea and other stomach troubles, but I have no evidence on that score. However, I do know that a similar infusion was taken to relieve menstrual pains and to ease childbirth.

A decoction of the leaves (of the same strength as tea) was said to relieve a bad cough and other chest complaints.

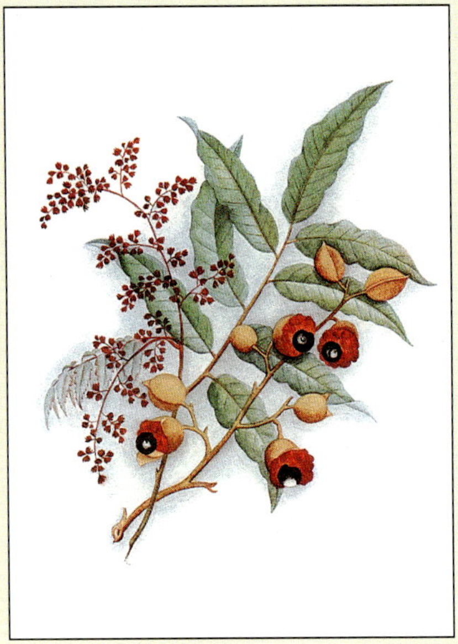

F. Osborne

Titoki

New Zealand ash

Alectryon excelsus

Titoki is a really fine tree found in both islands but particularly in Northland. In Kaikohe one street is lined with titoki and they certainly are an asset.

The black seed embedded in the red berry produces an oil which had many uses. For the oil to be extracted, the seeds were first placed in a strong bag of flax leaves then pounded with a club to bruise or smash them. The bag was then wrung out to extract the oil. This was applied to painful breasts as well as to sore eyes. It was also used for earache, especially in children. In earlier times Maori also used to rub the oil on their bodies to enhance their appearance.

The red pulp of the berry was also useful. An infusion of this provided another cure for blood spitting in people suffering from tuberculosis, and if a new-born baby's navel was inflamed a piece of soft cloth or scraped flax wrapped around the pulp was placed on it.

Toetoe

Cortaderia spp.

Cortaderia fulvida, C. *toetoe* and C. *splendens* are known to Maori as toetoe and are not to be confused with the introduced pampas grass that grows prolifically at roadsides. C. *fulvida* is generally found beside streams, while C. *splendens* is found on sand dunes and offshore islands. C. *toetoe* is found further south.

The top feathery part of the plant was applied directly to wounds to stop the flow of blood, and toetoe ashes were used to make a poultice for burns.

The sap of the lower part of the stem was applied directly to treat thrush in babies. I was told that chewing the young parts of the stem (young shoots) helped with diarrhoea. The pith of the lower stem boiled in water was used locally for kidney problems.

Toot, Tutu, Tupakihi

Coriaria arborea

Toot is a small-growing shrub found in most parts of New Zealand, especially in the North. It is a poisonous plant and affects cattle feeding on it.

The juice of the fruit was boiled with seaweed and the resulting jelly was much enjoyed as a delicacy by missionaries and children. It was also used for its mild laxative effect.

It is the external treatments, however, that I found most interesting. Shoots were scraped and heated for use as a poultice for bruises and flesh wounds. The leaves were similarly used, but first boiled until black. Sometimes all parts of the plant were boiled up and applied to wounds.

I had experience with 'football knees and ankles' (sprains), using poultices and the liquid. Results were remarkable. Players were active again within a week.

Toot was also prepared as a poultice for horse problems, such as sprains, cuts, and swollen joints. A friend of mine had a real difficulty with his horse. Someone had removed a gate at a gateway but not the gudgeons. When his horse passed through, it rubbed against the gudgeons and received a wound about a metre long and about seven centimetres deep. We made an infusion of toot leaves and bathed the wound, and then each day we removed the scab and bathed the wound. The shallow part healed within a week and the deeper part took about three weeks to a month to heal. A good horse was saved.

Totara

Podocarpus totara, P. cunninghamii

The totara is a tall tree found throughout New Zealand, and is perhaps the most versatile of our forest trees, with a soft wood suitable for carving yet durable for building, farm posts and strainers.

There are three totara species: the golden cultivar (*P. totara* 'Aurea') which we grow in our gardens, and the two common bush totara — *P. totara*, found in bush margins, on farms and lowlands, and the thin-barked totara, *P. cunninghamii*. *P. totara* has thicker, furrowed bark and smaller leaves than *P. cunninghamii*, which has more widely spaced leaves and is generally the species we see in the forest and at higher altitudes.

It is reported that Captain Cook had totara leaves infused as a drink for crew members affected by scurvy. The men found this unpalatable, so manuka leaves were added, which made the infusion more acceptable.

Maori boiled the leaves with manuka leaves and, after the liquid had been left for a week, it was taken as a drink to reduce fever. Paipai (a common skin disease) was treated by exposing the affected parts to smoke from burning totara wood. Women suffering from venereal disease were treated in the same way.

I have been told that an infusion of leaves rubbed on a bald head would promote growth of new hair. But, alas, I couldn't persuade any friends to try this.

Towai

Weinmannia silvicola

Towai or tawhero is found almost everywhere in Northland, in the forests and forest margins. It is very similar to the kamahi which generally grows further south (see illustration on page 78).

The inner bark was boiled in water and the liquid was used to treat cuts and burns.

The inner bark of kamahi was similarly prepared and the liquid used as a laxative and a strengthening tonic. I believe this decoction was also taken to relieve a cough.

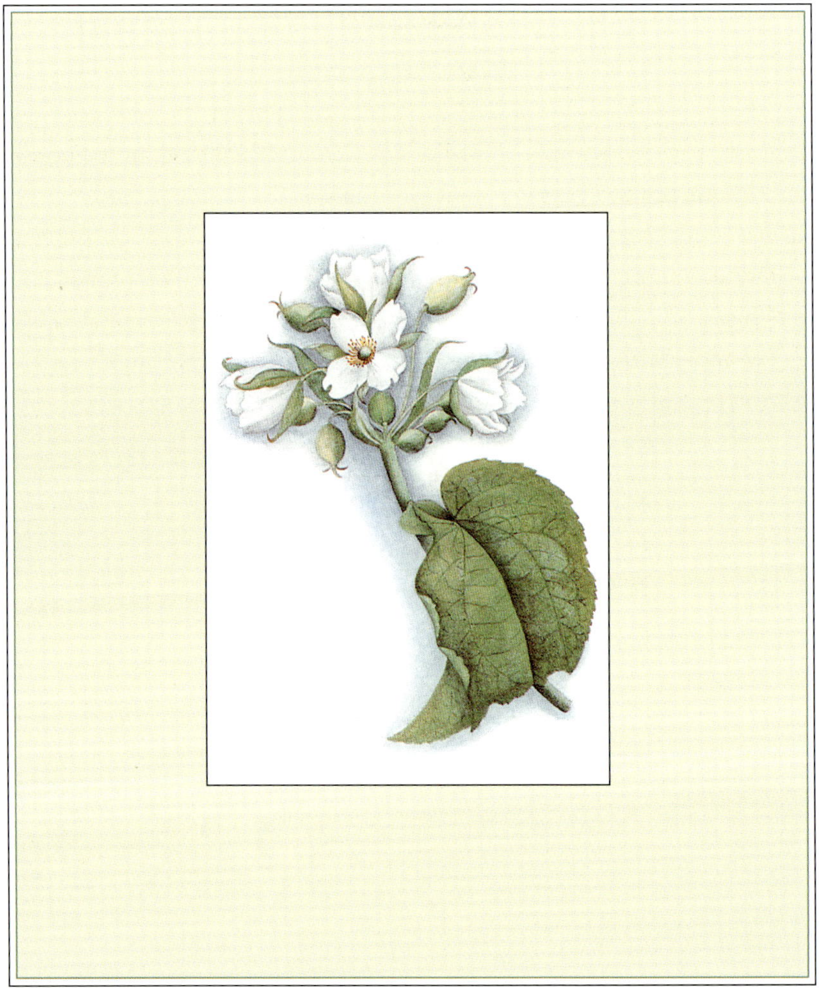

F. Osborne

Whau

Entelea arborescens

Whau is a lovely, broad-leafed shrub growing everywhere in the North, especially around Whangarei.

The leaves were heated in water and made into a poultice for treating wounds and sores.

Whau is so light that the stems were also used as floats for fishing nets, which were made from flax.

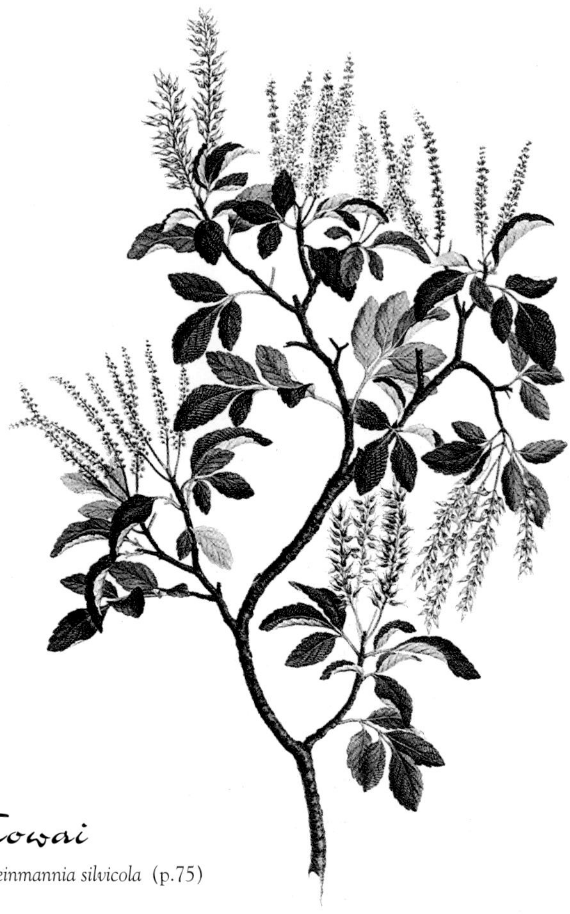

Towai

Weinmannia silvicola (p.75)

S. Parkinson
engraving

A Final Word

Dear Reader, take time off to walk the bush tracks, learn of our trees and plants, and you will be rewarded with the beauty and interesting detail of what you discover. Here I have only introduced the world of Maori medicine. A number of texts are available, however, that can provide more detailed information about the medicinal uses of New Zealand's native trees and plants.

Traditional natural therapies may enjoy a revival. When one considers, for example, that antibiotics today are needing to be stronger and stronger, there may come a time when they will have run their course. Will we return then to the natural medicines that I knew as a boy? Will young Maori start to use leaves, bark, roots, et cetera, in the same way as their elders? Perhaps lack of money will oblige them to try.

Will there also be greater research into the medicinal use of such native plants and trees as toot, karaka, and kowhai? More uses are already being found for manuka, poroporo and totara, and are proving very successful. It will be interesting to see what else develops in the future.

Recently a meeting of local people at my home decided to fence 80 hectares of the native bush reserve overlooking Kaikohe and the hospital, with the idea of eradicating possums, rats, stoats and weasels. We plan to plant more trees that the birds love, and you will find it will not be long before pigeons and tui come back. What a place to teach our young people about the beautiful trees that we have.